Talking with Your Physician by Lawrence W. Gold, M.D. Originally published April 2013 as I Love My Doctor, but...

A Grass Valley Publishing Production

Cartoons by Theresa Mccracken (mchumor@pioneer.net)

First edition February 2016

Printed in the United States of America

ISBN-13: 978-1523837250

ISBN-10: 152383725X

Dedication

To my wife, Dorlis

When I suggested my first non-fiction book, she was supportive, as usual, and said, "Go for it."

Acknowledgments

Dawné Dominique, a gifted artist and cover designer for help with the cover.

Donna Meares, editing.

Tony Lesce and Margaret Gold for their reviews and suggestions.

Theresa Mccracken, a gifted cartoonist who took my ideas and brought them to life.

Other Works By Lawrence W. Gold, M.D.

Fiction—Brier Hospital Series:

- First, Do No Harm
- No Cure for Murder
- The Sixth Sense
- Tortured Memory
- The Plague Within
- Trapped
- Hybrid
- Never Too Late
- State of Mind
- The Doctors' Lounge
- Out of Darkness

Other Novels:

- For the Love of God
- Rage
- Deadly Passage
- A Simple Cure

Non-Fiction:

Talking with your Physician (Surviving Obamacare)

All available in print, Kindle, and most as audiobooks.

Author's Note

If you're among the millions of patients who have a good relationship with your physician, this book may not be for you. In that case, you have my congratulations. Cherish and protect that association for the medicine of the future may make that relationshop increasingly problematic.

While I hope readers will enjoy this small book, it has serious intent as well. It deals with a pressing issue of our time, the provision of healthcare. The full implementation of the Affordable Care Act (ACA or Obamacare), makes this information even more important. The ACA is a compromise, perhaps the only one feasible for our times, but it's a troublesome one at that. I have hope that it will work out its bugs. As a more than satisfied Medicare recipient, I hope, some day, to see Medicare for all or its equivalent.

We're watching a war between two different approaches for paying for healthcare: government based and market based systems. Unfortunately, arguments about paying for healthcare have fallen smack into the political arena where ideology and power are more important than providing and improving care.

If we want to save money and provide good medical care, we should focus on the patient and his/her physician. Within that relationship is the pathway to providing healthcare that doctors and patients want, and society can afford.

This book may be more useful today than it was the first time I thought about writing it. I'd been thinking about how patients and their physicians got along, what's wrong with it, and how to make it better.

I've left the major healthcare issues for other's books (take your choice from the thousands). Providers, insurers, healthcare administrators, and politicians of every stripe have their own ideas about how to fix our healthcare system, but for the most part, they focus on how to pay for it.

I won't apologize for some repetitive material in this book because my aim is twofold: to educate and to persuade. The latter suggests coming at issues in different ways until I convince the reader to consider their value.

OBAMACARE

One wonders why the Affordable Care Act (Obamacare) that provides healthcare to millions lacking coverage, and eliminates major health insurance deficiencies, such as denying coverage for preexisting conditions, has been characterized as the most polarizing political legislation in decades. As Groucho Marx said, "Politics is the art of looking for trouble, finding it everywhere, diagnosing it incorrectly, and employing the wrong remedies."

Regardless of political persuasion, providing medical care to all who need it, via the Affordable Care Act or any other system, will result in exactly the same set of problems:

1. Many more people will require care:
   The ACA enrolled over eight million of which, over seven million are still subscribers.
2. More patients can overwhelm our already overburdened providers:
   Over 80 percent of physicians are overextended or working at full capacity.
3. More patient care in the face of uncontrolled healthcare inflation can stress or bankrupt the system or the individual: effective cost containment, an intrinsic part of the system, has yet to come to full fruition.
4. More patient care may not mean better care, in fact, it may make outcomes worse (see below).
5. Medical care is in transition to Accountable Care, a system to designed to reduce hospital admissions, specialty care, readmissions, and to encourage prevention. While these goals are laudable, elements may be destructive to the practice of medicine itself. Providers not meeting goals are guilty until they prove themselves innocent, choice suffers, and limiting referrals has the potential to harm patients.

The overriding message is: If you have a physician, make your relationship work for the both of you—you're in this together. If you don't have a physician, get one as soon as possible, but remember, you may be in trouble as even mediocre ones may be hard to find (See conclusions).

Personal Note

I've been a physician in the U.S. Army in Vietnam, private office and hospital-based practices, and have served as chief of a large department of internal medicine and family practice.

While from time to time, the media targets physicians for greed, mistakes, and attitude, still medicine scores high in surveys of the most respected professions, deservedly so, in my opinion. Largely, the physicians I've known rank high in those character traits people cherish the most: intelligence, dedication, honesty, and integrity.

Quotations

If you have more surgeons, you'll get more surgery. If you have more internists, you'll get more lab tests. (John Wennberg)

We shall have to learn to refrain from doing things merely because we know how to do them. (Theodore Fox)

Be careful about reading health books. You may die of a misprint. (or updated: may die of an Internet glitch) (Mark Twain)

I recently became a Christian Scientist. It was the only health plan I could afford. (Betsy Salkind)

According to a new report, more than 700 fake Obamacare websites have been created. Security experts say it's simple to identify the phony sites because they are easy to log on to.
(Jay Leno)

If you wouldn't want it done to you, don't do it to your patient.
(Lawrence W. Gold, M.D.)

The doctor is the only man who can suffer from good health.
(anon)

He is the best physician in whom, the patient has the greatest confidence.
(Peter Shaw

FORWARD

More than fifty years ago, in April of 1965, Dr. Morton Bogdonoff, the Chief Editor of JAMA, the Journal of the American Medical Association, wrote this abstract:

> During the past several years, one of the criticisms leveled at the practice of medicine in modern day America has been the supposed loss of the "old personal touch" from the doctor-patient relationship. These criticisms have been noted in both professional and lay publications, and have indicated that the blame is often leveled specifically at the increase in subspecialization, as well as at the use of complicated and intricate diagnostic procedures that entail much technical time leaving little for physician-patient interactions. Many of these communications have a tone of longing for the "good old days" and the physician of "horse and buggy" renown. Though the physician and patient may well have known each other much more intimately in years past, the "good old days" were perhaps not so "good," and one would hardly wish to return to a less effective type of medical practice.

Recently, I have spent time making rounds at a university hospital. While hospitals have streamlined their medical wards with computer systems that increase accuracy, deliver information rapidly, and keep track of diagnostic information, both current and past, my overall impression was not too dissimilar from previous experience. The intensive care unit had, in my day, acute care nurses at the bedside of the sickest patients. Today, however, nurses, physicians, and auxiliary medical personnel spend an inordinate amount of time before the computer, rather than at the bedside. This observation does not impugn the care they provide; it suggests that the current state of the art for the application of the computer to medical care has a way to go.

INTRODUCTION

If you trust Google more than your doctor, maybe it's time to switch doctors. (Jadelr and Cristina Cordova)

As if we don't have enough trouble in American life, economics, changing attitudes, and pressures suggest that it's time for us to deal with problems between patients and their doctors. It's easy to find guilt; just look at greedy doctors, ignorant and demanding patients, and the dysfunctional healthcare system. Oscar Wilde said it best: "It's not whether you win or lose, it's how you place the blame."

In addition, we have the Internet, a savior and a Pandora's Box (see computers in medicine).

The problems cited in this book are more than inconvenient or undesirable; they have a direct impact on both physicians and their patients. Specifically, these conflicts affect patients' lives, health, and—hold your hats, the cost of providing medical care.

Relationship (how I'm getting to hate that word) has become an overworked catchphrase. A Google keyword search on "relationship" produces over eleven million hits per month. Our major relationships, interpersonal, clergy, and with our physicians, have taken a hit, especially as we've seen patient-doctor relationships complaints increasing each year.

To paraphrase Shakespeare, the fault, lies not only in our HMOs, PPOs, or in the Affordable Care Act, but in ourselves. These systems don't make things any easier for physicians and their patients, but the need for medical care isn't going away, and most physicians still enjoy treating their patients. Improving medical care may be beyond the capability of our dysfunctional government and insurance industry, so, the trick, for the moment at least, may be to make do, or at least, not make things worse.

Often, it feels as if the world is conspiring against patients and physicians as politicians, insurance companies, and lawmakers complicate, confound, and challenge the relationship we'd all like to have with our physicians. I'm not talking about nostalgia for good times past where, for instance, the TV program *Medic* (1954-1956) opened with the announcer's dedication to physicians as, guardians of birth, healers of the sick, comforters of the aged…

The entertainment industry of the sixties and seventies produced the doctors we still yearn for today. The world (especially women) loved Dr. Kildare, Ben Casey, and Marcus Welby, but objective analysis of their behaviors would find them falling short in today's world, especially in their patronizing attitudes toward women. A 1971 Episode of Marcus Welby was entitled, "A Woman's Place…"

If you've lived long enough, you can remember the kindly, caring, self-sacrificing, humanistic, physicians who were unfailingly compassionate. How many physicians today live up to that ideal or even want to?

In May of 2007, Donna Karen wrote in the *Huffington Post*: Where is Marcus Welby, MD?

Nostalgia is great, but it won't get us the care we deserve, and it won't satisfy physicians who, even today, despite barriers, still thrive on helping their patients.

THE PROBLEMS

- Unrealistic expectations on all sides.

- The logistics of being a patient or a doctor.

- Malpractice litigation.

- Demands of healthcare insurers.

- Destructive attitudes:
    - Physician towards patient.
    - Patient towards physician.

- The almighty dollar (too much or too little).

- The profit motive in healthcare.

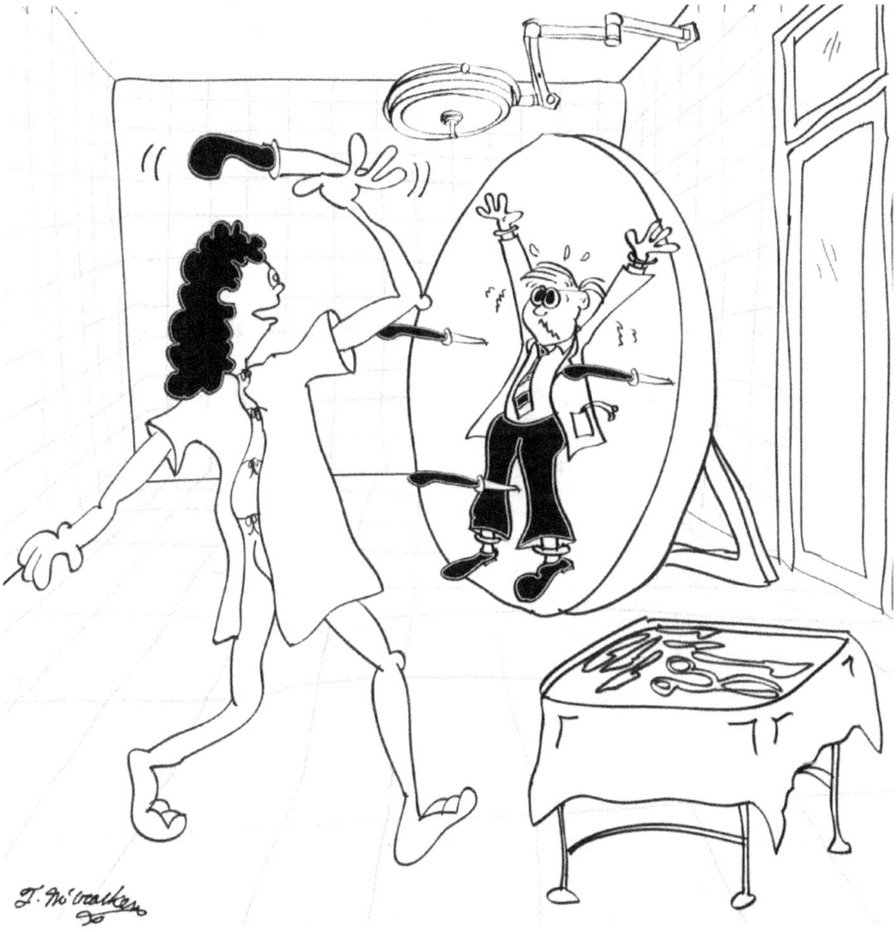

"THIS WILL ONLY HURT FOR A MOMENT."

I HATE DOCTORS NARRATIVES

(How can you fix a problem that you don't understand)

My doctor is nice; every time I see him, I'm ashamed of what I think of doctors in general. (Mignon McLaughlin)

I shouldn't have been surprised, but I was. Below are representative results of an Internet search on the phrase, "I hate doctors."

While I, and most physicians would find these examples unrepresentative and dismiss them, these comments, while extreme, intemperate, inaccurate, or just plain nuts, suggest that we would be smart to focus on their factual and emotional content, and ask, as they do in women's magazines, "Can this relationship be saved?"

If you're a physician, your reaction to these narratives will be similar to mine, but these opinions exist, and to some, they reflect a subset of reality.

These narratives are selected from actual comments on the Internet. I've partially edited, and paraphrased them to protect the innocent/guilty:

NARRATIVE I

I hate doctors because they do not care about what happens to their patients, they do not listen to their patients, they are rude, they pretend they are better than their patients, and they do not care about their patients' concerns. It is difficult to feel any kind of respect for someone like that.

It's rare to find doctors who actually care and don't talk down to their patients and can help patients in a meaningful way. I have never met a doctor who took feedback as an indication of how they were doing with their patients. Most interpret constructive criticism as a complaint or a threat. That puts them on the defensive and deprives them of a reality check on how they're practicing. It should be a wakeup call that has the potential to make them more humane since they are, in essence, heartless, soulless, cold, calculating creatures.

NARATIVE II

I can't express how much I hate doctors. The only time I will see one is when I am absolutely forced to, and only when someone else will pay the bill.

Every illness I have ever suffered cost me thousands of dollars in tests and doctor visits. First, they always keep me waiting, and afterward, they bounced me from one specialist to another at the cost of thousands more. I think they conspire with each other. Besides not listening, they don't believe what I say. Can you imagine how that feels? In the end, it's always a disease that any first year medical student could have diagnosed in thirty seconds.

Comment

Before we reject these critical observations as out-to-lunch, we should review objective studies of patient satisfaction where we will find, without the vitriol, some interesting correlations. Overall, complaints against physicians are up by 23% plus, mostly against general practitioners and psychiatrists.

Note that while complaints (gripes may be a better word) are more common against family practitioners and psychiatrists, lawsuits are more common against neurosurgeons, cardio-thoracic surgeons, general surgeons, family practitioners, and pediatricians (in that order). While it's clear that surgeons deal with higher-risk patients and worse outcomes, other factors may come into play such as more dramatic bad outcomes, easier prosecution, deeper pockets, and the tendency of malpractice insurance companies to settle claims.

In rough order of frequency, these are the complaints:

1. Waiting too long to get an appointment for an office visits.
2. Too much time sitting in the waiting room.
3. Physicians spent too little time with patients and didn't explain enough.
4. Didn't call with test results or return phone calls,
5. Lacked compassion.
6. Showed disrespectful and rude behavior.
7. Didn't listen to their patients, especially regarding what they've learned from reading, talking to others, or from the Internet.
8. Don't believe their patients or worse, think they're nuts.
9. Take your choice: The physician refers too often or too rarely.
10. Doctors disdain non-traditional medicine. They think they know everything.

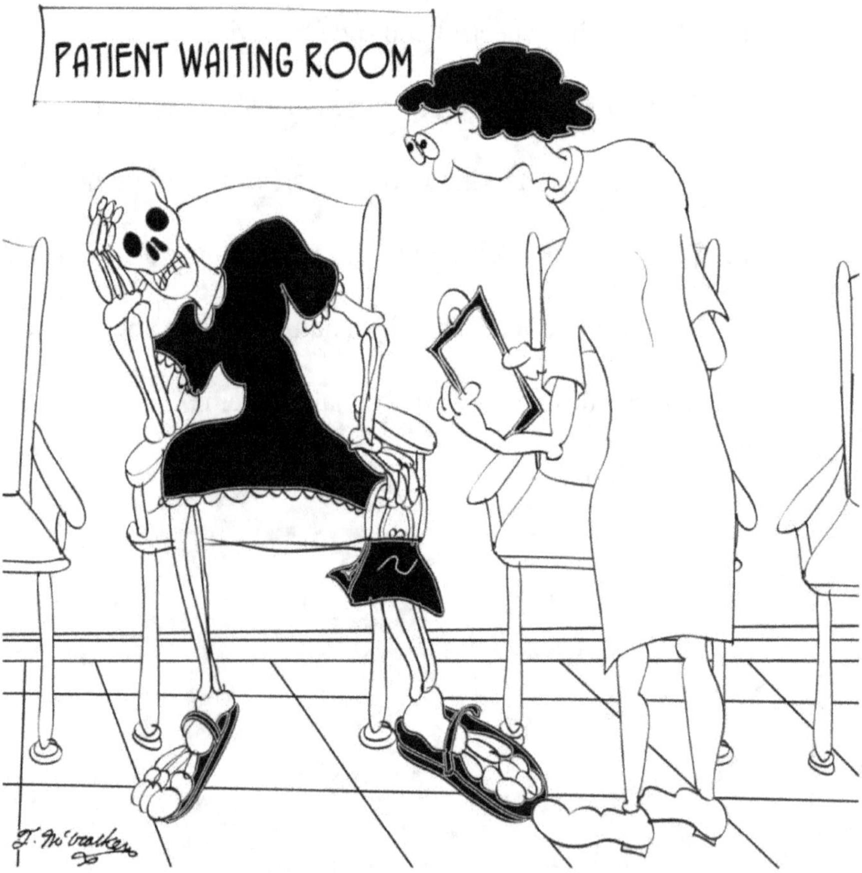

"DOCTOR WILL SEE YOU NOW."

PATIENT AND PHYSICIAN COMMUNICATIONS

THE CORNERSTONE OF MEDICINE

There is only one cardinal rule: One must always listen to the patient.

Oliver Sacks

An old joke about communications and medical language helps make the point:

Doc, says Steve, "I want to be castrated."

"What on earth for?"

"It's something I've been thinking about for a long time. If you don't do it, I'll just go to another doctor."

"OK, but it's against my better judgment."

Steve has his operation. The next day he walks down the hospital corridor very slowly, legs apart.

Heading toward him is another patient walking exactly the same way.

"Hi there," says Steve, "It looks as if you've just had the same operation as me."

"Yeah," says the patient, "I finally decided I'd like to be circumcised."

Steve's eyes widen in horror, "Oh no! That's the word!"

Doctors and Patients Don't Know How to Talk with Each Other

Even before we had the data, both physicians and their patients knew intuitively that communication between them was important. Clinicians, epidemiologists, university medical programs, and patient advocates filled the medical and general literature with studies describing the relationship, its deficiencies and recommendations for improvement.

Today, we know without question that better communication leads to more physician and patient satisfaction and improved outcomes. These outcomes, for example, include better control of high blood pressure, improved glucose control in diabetics, and less frequent episodes of asthma and congestive heart failure. A word before we get into communications: the medical literature contains many references to patient compliance or non-compliance, that is, how well patients follow their doctor's instructions.

Compliance, like the word tolerance, carries unintended meanings. When I hear of religious tolerance, for instance, it registers in my head as 'put up with' and when physicians talk about compliance, it suggests a subservient relationship between the patient and the physician. Synonyms aren't much better: accede, acquiesce, cave in, come around, consent to, and my all time favorite, cry uncle. Well-meaning healthcare advocates have even suggested the word concordance, but to my ears that sounds like an edict from the pope.

Let's give "adhere to" a shot. Substitute "comply," if you must.

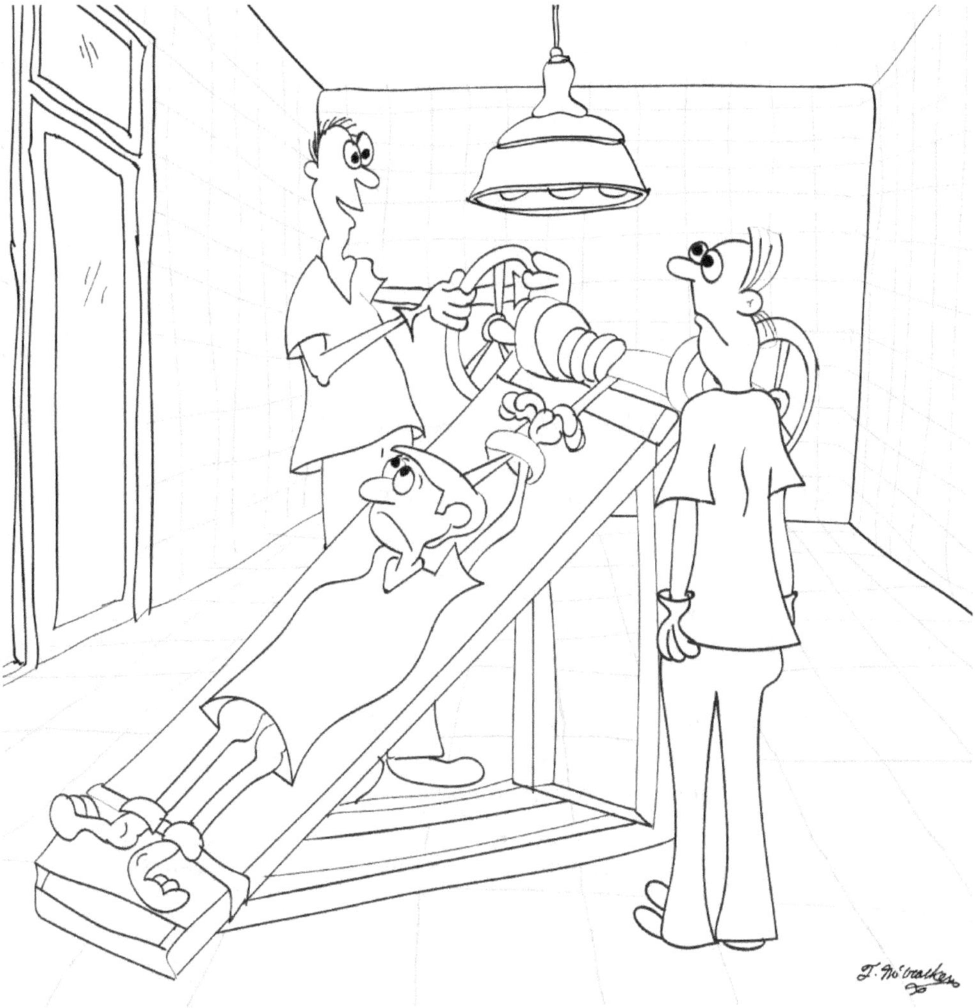

"I DON'T KNOW WHAT YOUR PROBLEM IS.
MY PATIENTS ALWAYS FOLLOW MY ORDERS."

Good communications leans to:

- Office visits are less threatening and more pleasurable for patient and physician.
- Diagnosis improves.
- Treatment is appropriate to the patient's condition.
- Adherence to recommendations for treatment and/or medications improves.
- Outcomes improve.
- Malpractice claims lessen.
- Physicians practice less defensively.
- Physician and patient frustration in the face of difficult medical problems are lessened.

While it's clear that these are qualitative improvements for docs and their patients, the economic impact is equally clear. For instance, sources estimate that non-adherence to physician recommendations costs somewhere between $100 billion and $289 billion dollars each year and results in 10 percent of hospital admissions. (The Atlantic Sept. 11, 2012)

Think of the human cost as well

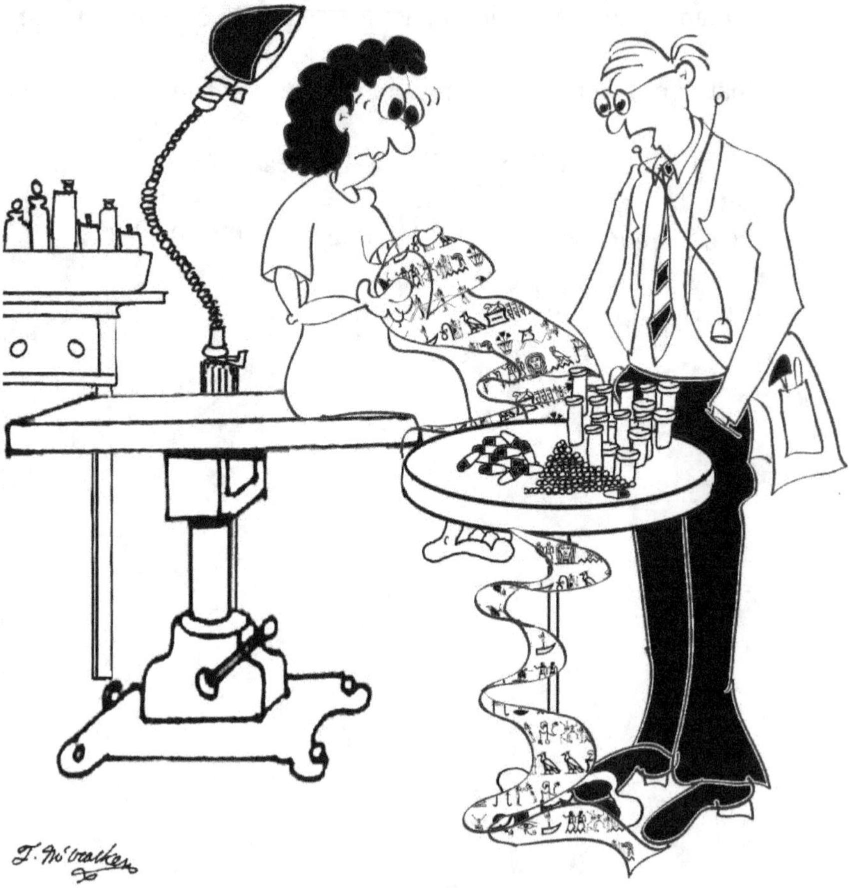

"JUST FOLLOW THESE SIMPLE INSTRUCTIONS."

Whose Life is it, Anyway?

Speaking up to your physician and/or following his/her recommendations are the most important things that patients can do for their health and well being. Yet getting some patients to speak up and comply is difficult to impossible. It's the equivalent of physician education: those who need it the most, shun it. Statistics are dismal and depressing for physicians who care about their patients. The remedy is beyond the scope of this work—maybe beyond the scope of any work.

The logic, however, is unassailable for patients and suggests conclusions most people would denounce: Is it possible that patients:

1. Don't care whether they're healthy or sick, or
2. Don't care if the live or die, or
3. Don't believe that medicine helps, or
4. Believe medicine helps, but it's not worth the effort, or
5. Exhibit denial, fear, anger, anxiety, loss of face and/or distrust of medical professionals? Factors that leave them paralyzed, or
6. Suffer from dementia or other mental illness, or
7. Can't decide which doctor, relative, or friend to listen to, or
8. Think the cost is too high, or
9. Can't tolerate the side effects, or any combination of the above.

Conversations with Patients

What's it like on the other end of the stethoscope!

Jacob versus a challenging patient

Jacob Weizman, the octogenarian physician in my novel, *No Cure for Murder*, is an experienced practitioner with great people skills and classical Viennese charm. Although at times abrupt and demanding, he cares for his patients as a loving grandfather. The patients in his practice return the affection. Even Jacob, however, can have trouble with a few patients:

"Who's next?" Jacob asked as he returned to his office from lunch.

Margaret, his office manager, stared at Jacob, guided him into his office, and sat with him on the sofa.

"With this prolonged prelude," Jacob says, "this next patient must a doozy."

"Amanda Koch has been a patient in at least ten East Bay practices, and for one reason or another they discharged her or she left on her own volition."

"Oh, I can't wait."

Margaret smiled. "It gets worse. She's sued several of our top docs and has submitted complaints against others to the Medical Board of California, or did both."

"I'm waiting for the punch line. There must be a reason why you're willing to subject us to this troubled woman. After all, we're supposed to be friends, right?"

"Ross Cohen, your favorite psychiatrist, thought that you might be the one to deal with her; that's a great compliment."

"Compliment," Jacob laughed. "That reminds me of the Phyllis Diller joke: You know you're old when someone compliments you on your alligator shoes, and you're barefoot."

Margaret laughed. "Still can't take a compliment."

"Ross can keep his compliments. I'll settle for peace and harmony. I've earned it after nearly sixty years practicing medicine." Jacob paused. "Okay. Do we have her medical records?"

"No. She doesn't want you biased against her even before you meet."

"Now, I really can't wait."

Margaret stood, left the room, and returned with Amanda. She was in her early forties with a stocky build and a bulldog demeanor. She had aggressive, spiky, and prematurely graying hair.

Jacob stood to greet her and offered his hand. "Jacob Weizman. It's a pleasure to meet you."

Amanda ignored Jacob's hand and plunked herself into the chair before his desk. "That's a bullshit way of starting this interview."

Jacob smiled. "Who's interviewing whom?"

"If I know anything about this medical community, you're welcoming me like the plague."

"I hate to burst your bubble, Ms. Koch, but until Margaret introduced us, I'd never heard your name."

"Call me Amanda." She paused. "And how did you know it wasn't Mrs. Koch?"

Jacob grinned. "A wild guess."

Amanda barely contained a small smile. "You're wondering why I didn't bring my records?"

"I assume that you didn't want me to see them—at least for now."

"I don't want the crap in those records to bias you, Dr. Weizman."

"You enjoy using salty language, Amanda?"

"I enjoy unambiguous language, Doctor. Does that offend you?"

"Absolutely not. It's better to know what's on a patient's mind than to guess." He paused. "I do need to know our objectives today so I can determine how to proceed. If you're auditioning me to provide medical care, then within my time limit today, let's get to it. If you've already decided to join this practice, then we need to get started with your history and a physical examination."

"What if I'm not ready to decide?"

"That's fine by me. I'll get paid for my time either way."

"That's all you guys ever think about."

"You don't know me well enough to say that. I could have retired many years ago, but I love practicing medicine and still have much to offer to my patients. Can I ask you a question or two?"

Amanda straightened up in her chair and tugged on her skirt. "Shoot."

"Are you happy with your relationships with physicians, and if not, how would you fix it?"

"That's a bit disingenuous, Doctor. You know my interactions with physicians have been disastrous."

"I don't care about the past, Amanda, as long as you don't paint me with the same brush. I don't care who was right or wrong, or who did what to whom. I'm not interested."

"Okay, but this sounds too good to be true."

"I've been around for a while, Amanda. I've seen just about everything one can see in medical practice. I promise to do the best I can and I'll always be honest with you. Do I enjoy practicing with the threat of malpractice litigation or a report to the medical board hanging over my head? Of course not, but you too will find that I have my own demands—reasonable ones, I assure you. We'll deal with them at the appropriate time, and you'll go along with them or move on to the next physician on your list."

"I have my own demands as well, Doctor… or can I call you Jacob?"

"Maybe when you get to know me better," he smiled. "Now, unless I'm mistaken, we'll continue our jousting, and we'll get to business on your next visit, if you choose to return."

"Okay, Doctor. Read 'em and weep. First, I'm no dummy, and if you treat me like one, we're going to have problems. I'm demanding and I want to know everything about my care. I'm a whiz on the Internet, and I'll know more about certain things than you do. If that threatens you, you'll just have to get over it."

"Anything else?"

"Yes. If you or someone in your office hands me a Patient's Bill of Rights, I'm gonna puke."

"Feels good, doesn't it, Amanda?"

"Why, yes it does, Doctor."

They bantered a while. "That's it for today," Jacob said. "I'll get you scheduled for the next available slot. I will have your medical records by then or you'll bring them with you." Jacob stared at Amanda. "It's been a plea…"

"A pleasure, Doctor?"

"It's been interesting meeting you, Amanda."

"Don't disappoint me, Doctor."

"Don't disappoint me, either, Amanda."

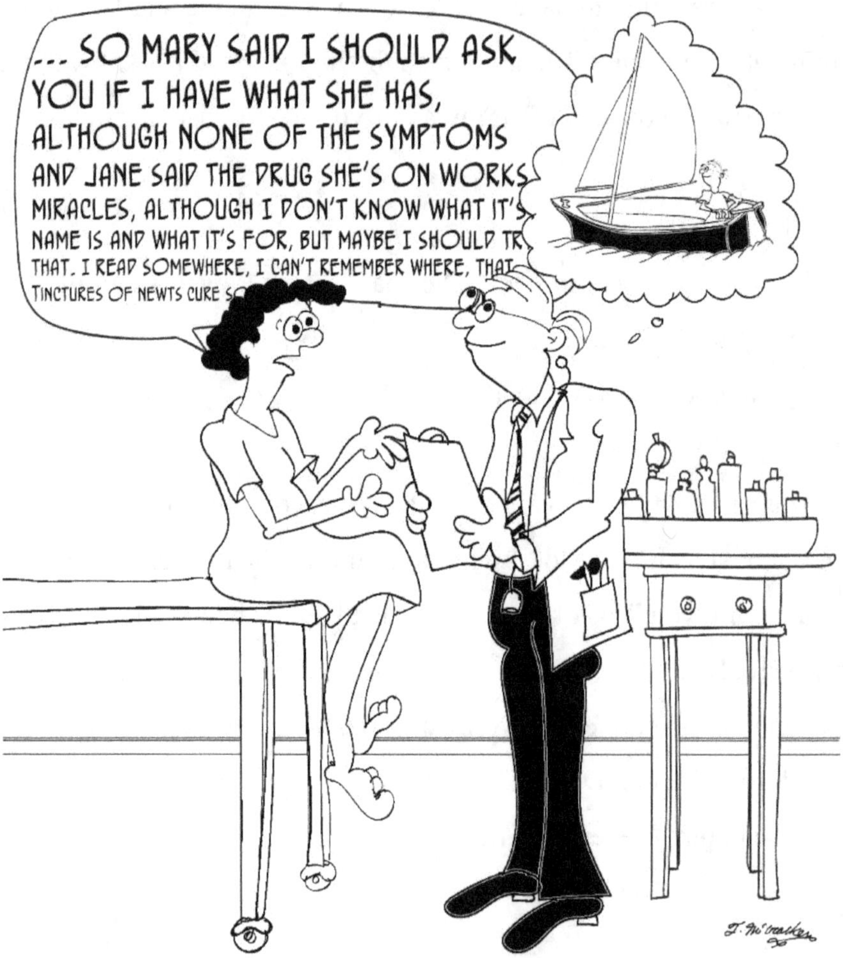
... SO MARY SAID I SHOULD ASK YOU IF I HAVE WHAT SHE HAS, ALTHOUGH NONE OF THE SYMPTOMS AND JANE SAID THE DRUG SHE'S ON WORKS MIRACLES, ALTHOUGH I DON'T KNOW WHAT IT'S NAME IS AND WHAT IT'S FOR, BUT MAYBE I SHOULD TR THAT. I READ SOMEWHERE, I CAN'T REMEMBER WHERE, THAT TINCTURES OF NEWTS CURE

QUESTIONS FOR PHYSICIANS AND PATIENTS

In regards to health, we expect physicians to answer our health-related questions. Patient answers to physician questions are to one extent or another optional due to issues of privacy. As you'll see from the physician questions below, privacy and the omission of essential medical facts may come at a price.

Tough questions for your Physician

If you're comfortable with your physician, asking questions and stating your concerns will be easier. Doctors and patients need to get along. Both share that responsibility and should use the same skills they employ in developing a successful relationship with friends, family, and colleagues.

If your physician is not open and available for reasonable questions, find another physician.

Samples questions/comments (for reference only).

No patient will ask the majority of these questions, nor should they. Physicians will often feel as if they're undergoing an interrogation if asked too many. Some questions are innocent and reflect a patient's needs. Others may come across as hostile, so don't ask them unless you are comfortable doing so, and you have reason to believe that your physician won't be offended. Nevertheless, keep them in mind and choose the ones appropriate to your situation and your concerns.

1. I didn't understand what you just told me. Please try again.
2. What's my diagnosis? What caused it?
3. How sure are you of my diagnosis?
4. Is this treatment or drug necessary?
5. How does the treatment work?
6. How will I know that the medication or treatment is working?
7. What are the risks and side effects of these medications?
8. Are generic medications okay?
9. What about medication purchased from other countries?
10. What about alternative medical treatments?
11. Are there treatments that don't involve medication?
12. How much will the treatment cost? Will my insurance pay?
13. What's my prognosis? Should I go to work on my bucket list?

14. Is it too late to start ballet or piano lessons?

15. How long will it be before I feel better?

16. If this treatment doesn't work, or I can't tolerate it, are there others?

17. Are you treating one problem or multiple problems?

18. What's the best time to catch you if I have questions?

19. What can happen to me if I refuse treatment?

20. What symptoms or signs should I watch for? Which ones require me to seek immediate care?

21. Should I see a specialist?

22, Are there clinical trials for my problem?

23. How do you justify so many tests?

24. (for women) Can I still have children? Can the medicine affect the baby?

25. Do you have a financial interest in medical, laboratory or diagnostic facilities?

26. How many operations of this type have you done?

ESSENTIAL QUESTIONS TO BE ASKED OF PATIENTS

(Questions that physicians should ask, but often don't)

These are serious, but sensitive questions and the physician should prepare the patient for their frankness. The physician needs to tell the patient that the practice asks these questions of everyone, including the clergy and little old ladies. The patient has the right to refuse to answer any and all. The Frustrated Physicians of America (FPA) has recommended polygraphs or lie detectors, but I do not advise them.

1. Did you understand what I said? Can you paraphrase it?
2. Do you want another opinion?
3. Should I explain this to your wife, mother, father, friend, etc.?
4. Do you want written information or references (links)?
5. Do you use street drugs? What kind? How much? How often?
6. Do you use (overuse) prescription drugs? What kind? How much? How often?
7. How much do you drink? How much? How often?
8. Have you suffered complications from drinking to excess? Blackouts? Tremors?
9. Have you been or are you now the subject of sexual/spousal abuse?

10. Are you having any problems with your sex life?
11. What is your sexual orientation? What specific behaviors? (esp. risky ones)?
12. Have you ever sued a physician for malpractice?
13. Have you had or are you having suicidal thoughts?
14. Have you had thoughts of harming anyone else?
15. Do you have trouble remembering things?
16. Do you regularly examine your breasts/testicles?
17. If you have guns in your home, are they properly secured?
18. Do you have an advanced directive for medical care?
19. Do you have a health directive? : It's appropriate at all ages beyond childhood as everyone is one accident or one severe illness away from needing one if you want your wishes fulfilled.

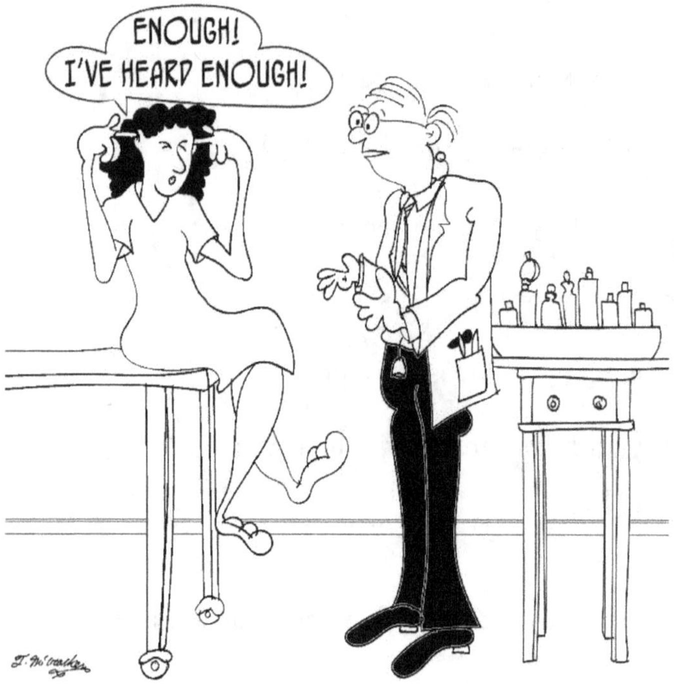
ENOUGH!
I'VE HEARD ENOUGH!

MEDICAL MALPRACTICE

While medical malpractice is not an intrinsically humorous subject, a little joke can't hurt. Physicians especially enjoy this one:

> A physician was browsing in an antique store when he came upon a statue of a rat. He asked the price and the owner said, "The statue of the rat is $100; the legend behind the statue is another $100."
>
> The man agreed to buy only the statue itself, although the owner warned as he left, "You'll be back for the legend!"
>
> The man tossed the statue into the back seat of his car and started to drive away.
>
> Several rats in a nearby alley began to chase the car. As he went through town, many more rats began to chase the car, until literally hundreds of rats were swarming the car.
>
> Frightened, the man sped toward the edge of town to a bridge over the river. He tossed the statue from the bridge and into the water below. All the rats jumped in after the statue and drowned.
>
> The man, now visibly shaken, returned to the antique store. The owner, seeing him approach, said, "Now, do you want the legend behind the statue of the rat?"
>
> "No," the man replied, "... but do you have any malpractice attorney statues?"

The unvarnished truths about malpractice suits

1. Most patients injured due to their doctor's negligence never file a lawsuit.
2. The risk of a malpractice lawsuit has little to do with the number of mistakes a physician makes.
3. A bad outcome doesn't indicate malpractice.
4. The best doctors are the ones sued more often.
5. Many of the worst doctors have never been sued.
6. Contrary to the urban legend of doctors protecting each other, the opposite is true. Doctors are responsible for 69 percent of malpractice lawsuits by advising the patients of other physicians to consult an attorney.
7. Thirty-eight percent of plaintiffs in malpractice cases are in the health profession.
8. Juries decide for the plaintiff in less that 10 percent of malpractice claims.

Malcolm Gladwell, in his book, *Blink* explains: Patients file lawsuits because shoddy medical care has harmed them—**AND** something else happened to them: They felt rushed, ignored, or poorly treated.

The Physicians' Guide for encouraging a malpractice claim.

Sue me, please!

1. Provide substandard care.
2. Spend as little time as possible with your patients.
3. Ignore or dismiss patients' observations.
4. Discourage patient participation in his/her own care.
5. Don't tell patients your plan for their care.
6. Blame greedy patients and greedier attorneys for malpractice claims.
7. Blame others, especially patients themselves for bad outcomes.
8. Refuse to explain medical mishaps.
9. Refuse to acknowledge actual losses, pain, suffering, and care needed in the future.

If a physician really wants to screw things up, he'll ask for the judgment of his/her peers since over 70 percent of those reviewing a malpractice claim are critical of the care provided by another physician.

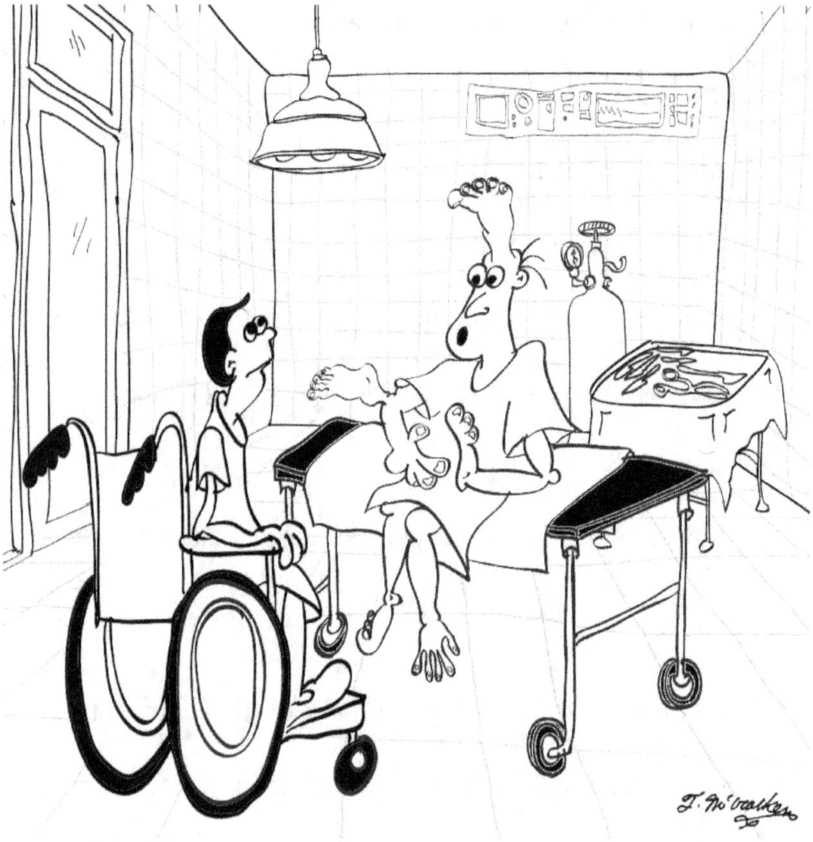

"THE DOCTOR WAS SO GOOD THAT I DIDN'T KNOW THAT IT WAS MALPRACTICE."

MATCHING PATIENT AND PHYSICIAN

(Love, hate, or indifference at first sight)

First Impressions: Physician-Patient relationships are more similar to how normal people get along than they are different. The charismatic Marcus Welby and Dr. Meredith Grey of Grey's Anatomy have **it**, whatever **it**, is. Patients love them at first sight, and often that initial infatuation outlasts reality and the trials and tribulations of medical care. Even when reality challenges belief, we still hear things like: Oh please! Marcus would never do that. Or, Meredith, she's the best, I never trusted anyone more. Even worse is; oh, you operated on the wrong kidney; no problem, Dr. Welby, I have another one anyway. Social scientists call this behavior cognitive dissonance, an explanation for why people fail to reevaluate first impressions despite evidence to the contrary.

Medicine hasn't quite gotten to a compatibility analysis equivalent to *eHarmony.com* yet, but we're coming to understand the principles that encourage good will and discourage discord.

Specialists in human relations have long believed that people make critical first impressions within two minutes, while others assert that it only takes thirty seconds. According to Malcolm Gladwell, in *Blink: The Power of Thinking Without Thinking,* the decisions may occur much faster, virtually instantaneously or in two seconds.

Most people swear by their first impressions and rue ignoring them.

First impressions are important—make the best of them.

A young doctor was just setting up his first office when his secretary told him there was a man to see him. The doctor wanted to make a good first impression by having the man think he was successful and busy. He told his secretary to show the man in. At that moment, the doctor picked up the telephone and pretended to be having a conversation with a patient. The man waited until the "conversation" was over. Then, the doctor put the telephone down and asked, "Can I help you?" To which the man replied, "No, I'm just here to connect your telephone."

Beyond First Impressions:

General Considerations:

An entire literature is devoted to the personality characteristics of physicians and patients and how well the different personalities work together. Like any generalization, it rarely applies to any specific pairing of patient and physician.

The patient's choice of a physician is much like matchmaking, but before getting into details, let me cite the **minimum** standards for choosing a physician:

1. He/she is competent.
2. Had good training at a reputable program.
3. Is on your insurance company's list of providers.
4. Has the experience you need in a physician.
5. Is the right age, sex, race, and ethnic background (no discrimination intended for patients are entitled to their choices, rational or not).
6. Is reasonably close to your home.

Beyond the bare minimum, studies show that patients want their doctors to be:

1. Confident
2. Empathetic
3. Humane
4. Personal
5. Forthright
6. Respectful
7. Thorough

Of course, you want to choose the best physician, but that choice is only step one. Developing a working relationship is equally or more important.

Physician Types

Type 1: Paternalistic, experienced, a sage: i.e. Marcus Welby.

Pros: Very comforting to patients. High trust and confidence are positive factors for wellness and improved response to treatment.

Cons: May not be best for patients who want to make their own decisions and/or rebel against paternalism.

Type 2: Authoritarian, dictatorial. Have strong bias toward their own beliefs. Tolerates little patient participation: i.e. Dr. Gregory House.

Pros: May have legitimate expertise to a patient's benefit. Putting up with this physician may be "worth it".

Cons: The belief in their talents may be overblown. Putting up with this physician may not be "worth it".

Type 3. A Partner in Crime, colleague.

Pros: Empowers patients. Will consider alternative treatments.

Cons: Leaves too many decisions to patient. Deprives patient the benefit of a physician's wider knowledge and experience.

Type 4. Counselor.

Pros: Will work with independent patients willing to make their own decisions.

Cons: Medical literature suggests patients using a counselor-type physician do worse with more medical problems and complications. (see below)

Type 5. Innovator.

Pros: Willing to try the newest therapy or drug.

Cons: Willing to try the newest therapy or drug. May become too enamored with new treatments to be objective.

Patients Types

Before people become patients, they're human, appealing or unappealing, kind or mean spirited, and accepting or rejecting. While the medical literature has tried to categorize patients, it may be better to focus on characteristics that earn some the title of "difficult patients". In an *Archives of Internal Medicine* article in 1999, authors found that physicians classified up to 15 percent of patient visits as "difficult." These patient types include:

- Dependent
- Anxious
- Demanding
- Manipulative
- Self-destructive

Instead, let's focus on patient *behavior* that physicians dislike. Many such behaviors are completely normal unless carried to extremes by patients who:

1. Bring in a five-page list of complaints.
2. Are rude.
3. Don't listen.
4. Constantly interrupt.
5. Fail to show appreciation for efforts of physician and staff.
6. Need constant reassurance.

7. Whose symptoms are never relieved by any treatment, or, if, relieved, the patients promptly develop new ones.
8. Are self–destructive.
9. Who threaten to or employ litigation against physicians.
10. Bring meddling and unhelpful companions.
11. Lie about their medication or their compliance.
12. Have no idea what medications they're taking.
13. Who take OTC medications or herbals and don't tell the physician.
14. Who stop their medications without telling the physician.
15. Reject lifestyle changes important to health such as exercise, smoking, drugs, and demand a pill instead.
16. Demand unneeded tests.
17. Demand unneeded medications seen in consumer advertisements.
18. Omit or delay reporting important symptoms.
19. Take medications from prior treatment or from a family member, especially antibiotics.
20. Demand medical excuse notes for work, school etc. without proper foundation.
21. Demand paperwork, forms etc. without appreciation of physician time constraints.
22. Seek drugs unrelated to true need, especially pain medication.
23. Who are excessively argumentative.

24. Who challenge physicians citing the Internet (Dr. Oz says…)
25. Make your own diagnosis and demand a specific treatment.
26. Ask another question just as doctor is leaving or say, "by the way, I'm having chest pain."

Phrases physicians hate:

1. It hurts all over.
2. I always get antibiotics for that.
3. I'm sensitive to all medication.
4. Medications don't work on me.
5. I lost my pain pills (or the dog ate them).
6. I don't believe you. Show me the study where…

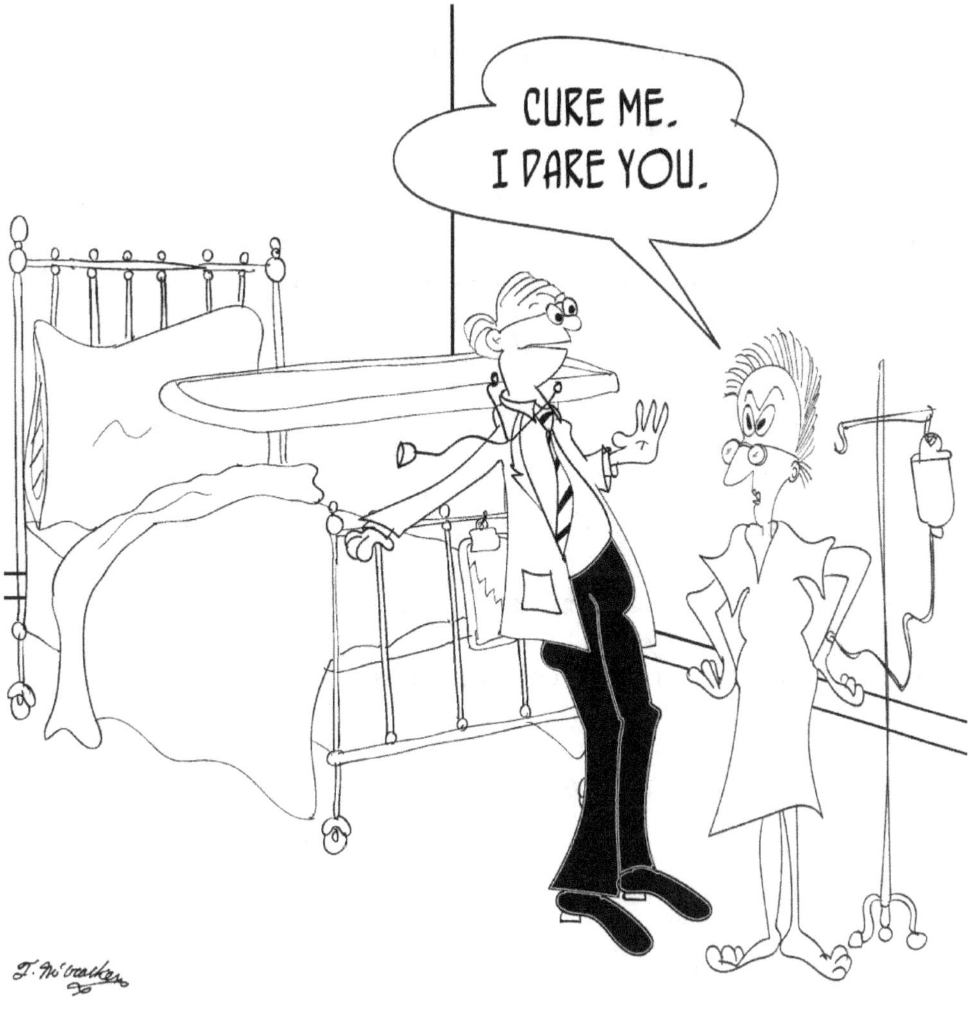
CURE ME.
I DARE YOU.

BE CAREFUL WHAT YOU WISH FOR

Giving patients exactly what they want, versus what the doctor thinks they need is proving to be bad medicine. Researchers at UC Davis studied data from a large number of patients and found that the most "satisfied" patients:

- Spent more on health care and drugs.
- Were 12% more likely to require hospitalization.
- Accounted for 9 percent more in health care costs.
- Were more likely to die.

The reasons for these outcomes are complex, but research does show these patients receive more discretionary services, use more drugs (with side effects), and undergo more procedures (with their risks).

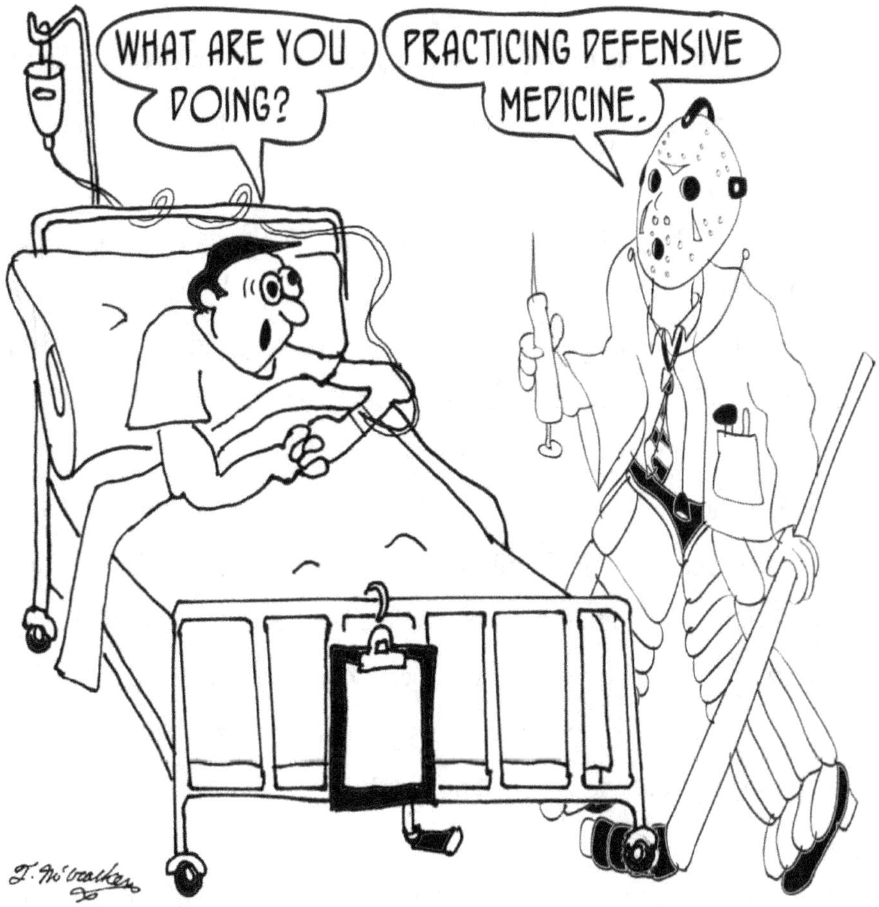
WHAT ARE YOU DOING?
PRACTICING DEFENSIVE MEDICINE.

THE "MORE IS ALWAY BETTER" PHILOSOPHY

In a world of limited resources, why would we want more done to us, especially when doing more leads to worse outcomes?

The answers are simple:

Patients demand more as they equate more with better care.

Reimbursement systems encourage the physician to do more. Do more; get paid more.

The threat of malpractice litigation demands the physician do more for self-protection.

Health care management systems are increasingly using patient satisfaction (or doing more) as an index of physician performance.

Patient satisfaction is becoming the siren song for providing health care and the Achilles heel for those who embrace competition as the savior for our costly system. It's perfect; patients get more, doctors get more, and health management systems glow with competitive nirvana. Everything's fine until we discover that the costs are increasing, patients are doing worse, and finally, we're running out of money—then what?

It's beyond the scope of this booklet to get into more detail on this complicated issue, except to remind the reader that doing more can have significant downsides for the patient and the system.

MEDICAL PROBLEMS THAT PHYSICIANS DISLIKE

While Marcus Welby may feel unqualified love and acceptance for all his patients, real physicians find dealing with certain medical conditions more problematic. If you are a patient with one of these conditions (see below), and entitled, like everyone else, to treatment, it's better to know this up front in order that you and your physician can work together.

Even when patients and physicians act in good faith, certain medical problems frustrate both patient and physician because:

1. Treatment is inadequate or incomplete.
2. Non-adherence to treatment is high.
3. Diagnoses may be uncertain.
4. The problems tend to recur.
5. They impact on the patient's social skills creating difficulty for physicians (it's difficult to be cheerful and outgoing when you don't feel well). It's too easy to blame the physician.
6. A physician's failure to treat or control a disease is frustrating. It's too easy to blame the patient.

These disliked diagnoses include:

1. Obesity.
2. Alcoholism/substance abuse.
3. Anxiety/depression (what we previously called 'neurosis').
4. Psychosomatic illness.
5. Chronic pain disorders.
6. Incompletely understood diagnoses such as fibromyalgia and chronic fatigue syndrome.
7. Chronic illnesses, in general.

Effective strategies exist for patients and physicians in dealing with these illnesses, but patients should know up front that it ain't easy. Putting out a contract on such patients is a common suggestion, but it's probably not advisable (although, as a consultant, it may generate more referrals).

FINDING A PHYSICIAN

(The right physician)

In the best of worlds, we'd have our choice of physicians. Today, unfortunately, many parts of the country have too few physicians, physician have limited their practices because of volume or their refusal to accept some insurance plans (See Obamacare comments).

That doesn't mean that you need to accept any physician willing to open their practices to you. In small towns, with limited numbers of physicians, or in large cities with practices that are full, patients face difficult and uncomfortable choices. How can no care be better than any care? Patients and families must simply do the best they can, but if possible, don't take the easiest way.

Advice About Finding a Doctor

Select a physician before you need one.

- BEST: Have a physician you trust refer you to a specific physician/specialist.
- Choose from among friends and associates those most intelligent, critical, and demanding, and solicit their opinions.
- Manage to have a doctor in your family, especially one you love and trust. Get his/her opinion.
- Find a way to meet with a nurse working in a hospital. Nurses know who the best doctors are. Be careful about asking hospitals, medical societies, or physician networks for referrals, as they're likely to send you to practices needing patients. There may be a reason why practices need patients (doesn't apply to new practices).
- Check with the state licensing division regarding complaints against a physician.
- Sit down with a prospective physician. Good first impressions may not guarantee a perfect match, but bad impressions surely do. Trust your gut.
- If the waiting room is filled with unhappy people growing old from waiting, think twice.

- Remember, you're not marrying a physician. If it's not working out, get a divorce.
- On-line rating services may help, but remember human nature; people are more likely to report fault than praise.

MEDICAL MYTHS

I'm including this section, not only because it's important, but also medical myths are a frequent source of conflict between patients and their physicians.

Few activities generate as much acrimony as challenging established beliefs. To the best of my knowledge and from the review of the literature, these myths cited below need debunking. Truth, however, is an inadequate defense against established belief. Psychologists and psychiatrists call that cognitive dissonance: the mental stress or discomfort experienced by an individual who holds or acts on two or more contradictory beliefs, ideas, or values at the same time. New information that conflicts with these existing beliefs, ideas, or values is especially troublesome.

Here are the myths, the common beliefs, and the information that contradicts them.

I'm girding myself for the torch and pitchfork crowd (patients and physicians).

MYTH #1: "Overweight" Means "Unhealthy"

One study tracked more than 25,000 men for over 23 years. They recorded who got sick and who died and who didn't. In the end, the study surprised the world by showing that men who were overweight or obese but exercised regularly had half the death rate of normal-weight men who were out of shape. In fact, the study found that being in poor physical condition was far more dangerous than simply being overweight, increasing the risk of premature death as much as having type 2 diabetes, high blood pressure or cholesterol, or smoking cigarettes does.

MYTH #2: Prescription Drugs Are Guaranteed Safe

With intense publicity, few still believe this myth.

About 10 percent of prescription drugs that hit the market are later discovered to cause serious side effects that didn't turn up in clinical trials.

MYTH #3: Hospitals Are Sterile Houses of Healing

According to the Centers for Disease Control and Prevention, 1.7 million people develop infections while staying in, or immediately following discharge from US hospitals each year. Nearly 100,000 die.

MYTH #4: Sleep Isn't That Important

It's nearly universally accepted that sleep is important at any age.

MYTH #5: The Placebo Effect Is Negligible

35 percent or more of test patients responded as though they had received real treatments. The placebo effect is so powerful that it's the reason we depend on double-blind clinical trials.

MYTH #6: Too Much Salt Is Bad For You

Based on some very weak studies fraught with uncertainty, salt has been blamed for a variety of medical conditions—resulting in calls for extensive reduction or even elimination of it in food products.

This is another misconception unless you are a specific genetically engineered lab rat. Normal kidneys can always clear salt except in specific medical conditions related to the kidneys, heart, or liver—for these, salt restriction is mandatory. In patients with high blood pressure, some are salt sensitive, others not. A recent study (this blows my mind) suggested that salt restriction may worsen the condition in those with congestive heart failure.

MYTH # 7: Ulcers Are Caused By Stress

Harmful stomach bacteria, rather an acid levels or stress, are in fact to blame for stomach ulcers. The H. pylori bacteria, believed to be spread via person-to-person contact, apparently weakens the mucus lining of the stomach, paving the way for stomach acid to attack our delicate stomach lining.

Myth # 8: Old People Sleep Less

It is often heard that the older you get, the less sleep you need. This myth couldn't be more wrong since it's the complete opposite.

Myth # 9: Chocolate causes Acne

There have been a lot of scientific studies that prove that there is little to no chance that chocolate or greasy food can cause acne breakouts.

Myth # 10: Resting for Back Pain

Studies have shown that patients that engage in regular activities tend to recover faster and have fewer problems with recurring pain.

Myth # 11: Over Exertion causes hearth attacks

Most believe that heart attacks can be caused by excessive exertion, and that rest and a more carefree lifestyle is necessary for recovery. But the surprise is that a less active lifestyle is more likely to cause heart conditions.

Myth # 12: Vaccines can cause developmental disorders in children.

This remains a hotly debated issue, despite being debunked in multiple large studies.

Myth # 13: Catching a Cold in Cold Weather (COULD YOUR MOTHER BE WRONG?)

People spend much more time indoors in cold weather closer to others. This makes it easier for the virus to spread.

Myth # 14: You Should Drink 8 Glasses of Water a Day (my wife and her friends are going to kill me for this one)

This one can be traced back to a 1945 recommendation from the Nutrition Council that a person consume the equivalent of 8 glasses of fluid a day.

Water may transiently make you feel full, but it has no other benefit.

If you're not thirsty, you most likely don't need that glass of water.

Myth #15: We use only 10 percent of our brains

Advanccs in mcdical tcchnology through the twentieth century have revealed this to be untrue, as imaging studies like MRI and PET scans clearly reveal that no area of the brain is actually dormant.

Myth # 16: Medical Diagnosis is always accurate

When you receive a diagnosis from a doctor, we aren't always 100% sure it is correct.

THE PROBLEMS WITH MEDICAL ADVICE

(INCLUDING MY OWN)

The most common misperception of all has to do with giving medical advice—after all physicians are in that business. What are the limits of such advice when we know from experience how poorly patients and even loved ones will follow recommendations? When we advise losing weight, getting exercise, stopping smoking, controlling a diabetic's blood glucose, taking medication, how much is enough? And when we advise patients to get the benefits of proven screening procedures such as mammograms, colonoscopies, and regular office visits, how many will comply?

Here are three alternative approaches:

1. Nagging: The pain-in-the-ass approach. Persist in giving advice although we know patients will not follow it.

2. Surrender: Have your say to the patient and fuggedaboutit—hell, it's their lives, after all.

3. Co-opt the advisee. The most difficult approach; urging without nagging, persisting without becoming obnoxious, and encouraging based on a scientific truth; that sincere attempts to change a behavior while failing over and over again, will ultimately succeed (if you both should live long enough).

INTRODUCTION TO MEDICAL TERMINOLOGY

What the heck is he/she talking about?

The Centers for Disease Control (CDC) estimates that 9 out of 10 adults have trouble following their physician's advice largely because they find it incomprehensible. Low health literacy leads to lack of appropriate treatment and poor adherence to recommendations, costing approximately $238 billion a year, and untold pain, suffering, and even death.

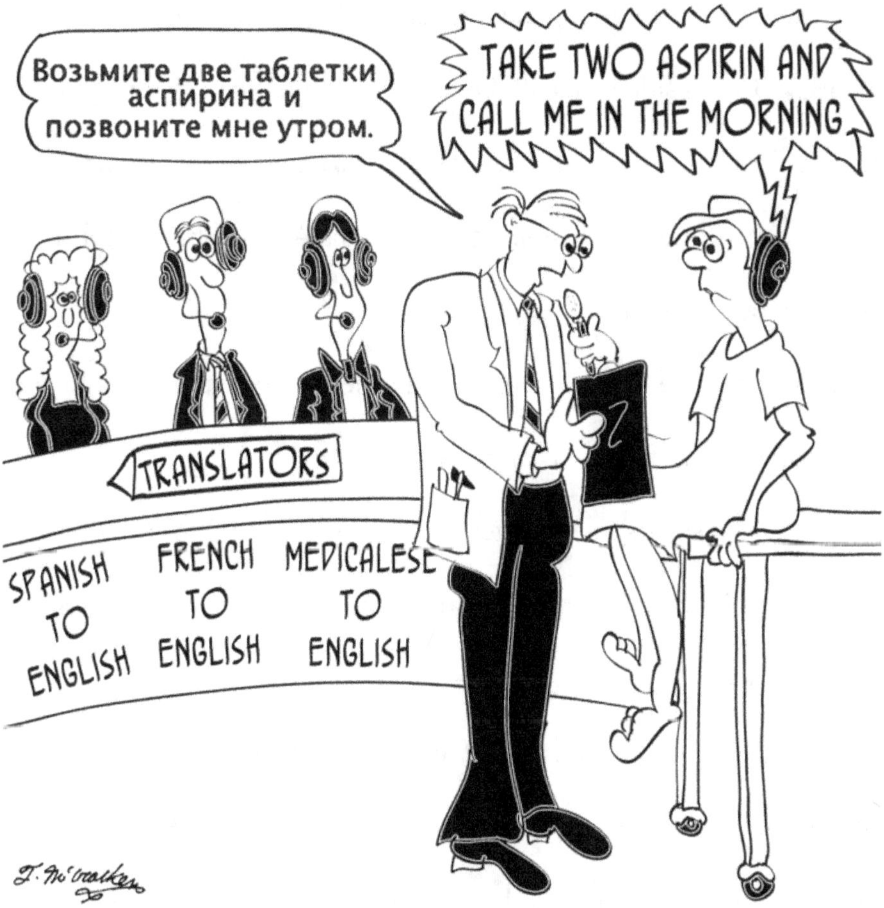

The reasons why patients don't understand:

1. Use of scientific jargon.
2. Confusing instructions from physicians.
3. Complicated medical phrases.
4. The healthcare provider doesn't have the time, or doesn't take the time to be sure that patients understand.

The move is on at all government levels to simplify language. Note that on October 13, 2010, President Barack Obama signed the Plain Writing Act of 2010 which requires the federal government to write documents, such as tax returns, federal college aid applications, and Veterans Administration forms in simple easy-to-understand language…"

At the present time, 2/3 of Medicaid agencies write health material at a reading level between fourth and sixth grades.

Despite the naysayers, medical terminology is essential for physicians, other health care professionals, and yes, that fact poses a problem for those outside the profession.

When a patient says, "I had a heart attack", the health professional is at a loss to understand. Did that patient have:

- A myocardial infarction caused by a blocked artery to the heart muscle, *or*

- An arrhythmia, an abnormal heartbeat, *or*
- Congestive heart failure, where the heart pump fails to keep up with the body's need for oxygen carrying blood, *or*
- Some other heart or lung event?

If the medical record is available, that can help, but often it's not or it's incomplete and leaves the medical staff confused or worse.

Medical terminology is not a conspiracy against patients, friends, and relatives. There are no physician black helicopters flying in to steal your Internet connection to *WebMD*.

Physicians use medical terminology because it's precise. If one health professional tells another that John Jones had a myocardial infarction, he/she knows exactly what happened.

In any case, patients, families, and others need to understand what's happening to them and to their loved ones. They're entitled to know, and it's the health care professional's responsibility to help them understand to the best of his/her ability. That means explaining medical terminology or using lay words. That may sound simple, but consider:

- Do physicians have enough time and patience?
- Do all patients want such detailed information?
- Will healthcare insurers allow the time needed for such explanations?
- How to explain to those unable or unwilling to understand?

COMPUTERS AND DOCTOR-PATIENT RELATIONSHIPS

In the United States approximately eighty-three percent of office visits include the use of the computer in the examining room. While physicians, patients, and healthcare systems laud computerization as a godsend to medical care, studies have raised questions about its overall effectiveness at this moment in time.

A 2013 RAND survey of physicians found mixed reactions to electronic health record systems, including widespread dissatisfaction. Many respondents cited poor usability, time-consuming data entry, needless alerts, and poor workflows. Entering and retrieving information into the computer can take a physician inordinate time compared to entering the information in a paper medical record. And, the high number of entry clicks can make physicians feel like data-entry clerks.

A recent *New York Times* article cited the following narrative: A friend of mine, a physician in his late 60s, recently described a visit to his primary care doctor. "I had seen him a few years ago and I liked him," he told me. "But this time was different." A computer had entered the exam room. "He asks me a question, and as soon as I begin to answer, his head is down in his laptop. Tap-tap-tap-tap-tap. He looks up at me to ask another question. As soon as I speak, again it's tap-tap-tap-tap." This patient's response—he changed doctors.

Computer errors, changes in workflow, and a huge number of false alarms have physicians longing for the good-ole-days of pencil and paper.

I'd spent a good deal of my professional career in intensive care units where nurses and physicians spent time in direct contact with patients. Now, they spend much time at the computer.

I do not doubt the potential benefits of computerization on patient care, but for the moment, we're in a transition zone, in computer terms—beta testing. Let's enjoy the obvious benefits, but remain diligent to the potential problems.

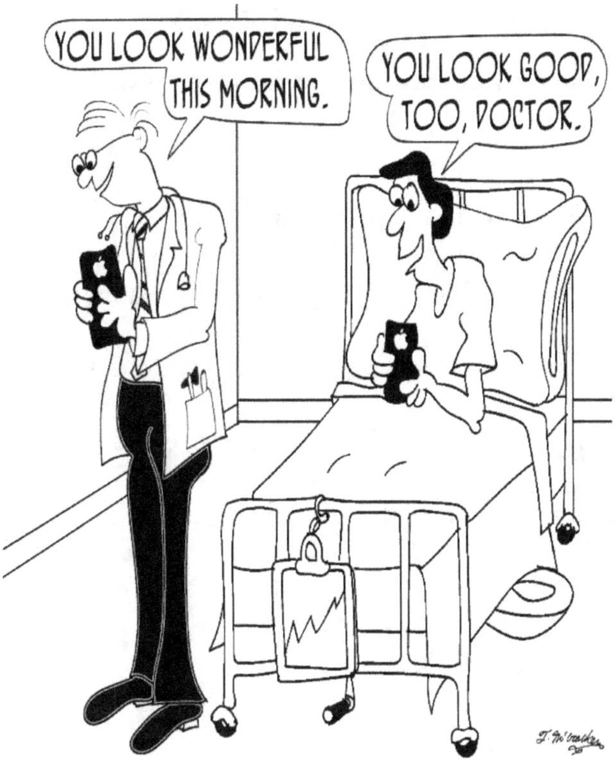

SUGGESTIONS

If you feel that the computer's getting more attention than you do, it won't be a surprise that your physician feels the same way. When he or she glances away from the computer screen, smile and ask, "Can I have a moment of your undivided attention?"

FINDING ANSWERS ONLINE

Research online, but do so carefully and only at respected web sites

Just because you read something on the Internet, does not mean it's true. If you want to search on specific diseases, diagnoses and treatments do not use Google or its equivalent. Such searches will produce a large number of hits, and many, perhaps the majority, will provide inaccurate or even dangerous information. It's better to search reliable sites that contain reputable information reviewed by experts.

- **http://www.mayoclinic.com**
- **http://www.cdc.gov**
- **http://www.fda.gov** (especially good for drug information)
- **healthfinder.gov**
- **http://www.medlineplus.gov**
- **http://www.webmd.com** (user-friendly site)
- **http://www.cancer.gov**

Be careful with sites claiming to provide accurate information about hospitals and physicians. Such evaluations are complicated and error-prone.

CONCLUSIONS

(Getting along)

In 1936, Dale Carnegie published *How to Win Friends and Influence People*. To date, its sales have topped 15,000,000—not bad for a sales representative for Amour and Company.

> To paraphrase his concepts, both patients and physicians should appeal to the other's highest ideals, speak in terms of the other's interests, and allow each other to save face by avoiding unproductive challenges. Common courtesy is the key and you're more likely to enjoy each other's company the next time you meet.

Altruism:

Patients have always taken physician altruism as a given. Sure, physicians have enjoyed status, privilege, and material and financial security, but at the core is the public's belief that their physicians are honest, have integrity, and act on behalf of their patients based on underlying altruism. As the public image and physicians' self-image declines with loss of status, privilege, financial security, and independence, what's left is altruism; hardly a sound basis for a career in our materialistic world. Our best and brightest are proving that by foregoing the M.D. for an MBA, advanced scientific degree, or heading to Wall Street or the boardroom, or Silicon Valley. In a quote from the prestigious British Medical Journal, "there is a growing feeling that altruism in medicine, if not dying, is at least declining."

Caring about others is not unique to physicians it belongs to patients as well. Its potential exists in all human beings, but too often, it remains dormant. Altruism may be the one mechanism remaining for patients and their physicians to change the system for the better. If not, the government, acting under the less than altruistic influence of politicians and lobbyists, will make the decisions about medical care for all of us.

HOW TO SAVE THE RELATIONSHIP WITH YOUR PHYSICIAN

(If you want to)

Competent and trustworthy physicians are hard to find.

If the patient-physician interaction becomes a power struggle, nobody wins. I never thought the day would come when I'd quote Republican Tea Partier, Jim DeMint, but wisdom exists independent of its source. He said: Compromise works well in the world when you have shared goals. I can see no better example than this relationship.

1. If you know which words will anger or alarm your physician, don't say them.
2. A pleasant and rewarding office visit today, increases the likelihood that they'll continue in the future.
3. Be as specific as possible when describing your problems. Vagueness not only makes a physician's job more difficult, it turns them off. Don't minimize your problems, especially pain.
4. If a physician does something extra for you or your family, acknowledge it. If it's obvious that the physician is particularly busy, acknowledge that, too.
5. Just because you're a big shot somewhere, don't act entitled with your physician.
6. Leave bad breath or body odor at home (unless they're the problem).
7. No thoughtful physician expects you to accept everything they say, but unless you have evidence to the contrary, give the physician the benefit of the doubt and keep an open mind.

8. If you have ten things you must discuss with your physician, start with the most important first.
9. If you have information about your illness to share with your physician from the Internet, the media, from other patients or physicians, don't present them as a challenge. A simple, 'this is what I heard—what do you think,' is reasonable.
10. If you're ethical, expect your physician to be ethical, too. Don't ask for false reports or unjustified excuses.
11. Complain about the physician's staff with care. After all, he picked them. If they deserve criticism, don't hesitate to voice your concern, but, if possible, bring it first to the office manager or head nurse.
12. Thoughtful physicians understand that certain people, through no fault of their own, don't get along. Be careful when you complain about previous physicians or consultants for the physician will think, *Am I next?*
13. Speaking up may be the most positive thing you can do for your health, as the American Society of Internal Medicine estimates that seventy percent of correct diagnoses come from information provided by the patient.
14. If you think that after a lifetime, you or your physician is going to change, think again. How about making the best of it?

WHEN SHOULD YOU FIRE YOUR DOCTOR

At first, I thought this section might be superfluous, as it represents the polar opposite of those thoughts incorporated in several preceding sections about patient/physician communication, but there's something about brevity and lists that catch a reader's attention.

Most patients are discomforted by the prospect of firing their physician, and while for most people, it takes dissatisfaction over a prolonged period of time to get to this point, many people do get that far. I have several suggestions:

1. Make sure that you have engaged the services of another physician first. This is especially important in an environment where the number of physicians is declining or you live in an area where many practices are full and not accepting new patients (i.e. Obamacare).

2. As many women's magazine have a section entitled, "Can this marriage be saved?" so, too, patients should consider whether or not they could save their relationship with their physician. Too often, the patient and the physician are misreading each other and ascribing unjustified motives to each other. A frank discussion, reality based, may resolve these issues or confirm the patients' suspicion that it's time to cut and run.

SIGNS SUGGESTING THAT YOU SHOULD FIRE YOUR DOCTOR

1. You just don't mesh. You dislike each other.
2. You dread coming to the doctor's office.
3. He doesn't respect your time or you feel rushed on each visit (you need to respect the doctor's time as well).
4. He doesn't explain herself or her recommendations. He prescribes medication without describing the reasons, her expectations, alternatives, and possible side effects. He doesn't interpret lab or other diagnostic tests. He uses too much jargon.
5. He doesn't listen to you or value your input. He doesn't show concern for your physical or emotional well-being.
6. He doesn't allow you to make the final decisions about your care or pressures you excessively.
7. He doesn't seem happy in her work.
8. Her office staff is unprofessional and/or disorganized.
9. Circumstances make you question her competence.
10. He acts on her own and doesn't coordinate with other physicians.
11. You can't reach her when you're ill or get an appointment in a reasonable period of time. "Doctor's too busy, go to the emergency room" wears thin if it happens too often (many caring practices manage to "squeeze" patients into a busy schedule when needed).
12. He's rude and/or condescending.
13. He doesn't understand that doing more, even at your insistence, may not help, and might make things worse.

Pay attention to unspoken messages and your own feelings. They are usually significant. It's difficult for a doctor to do her best, or a patient to benefit from care if they are not comfortable with their physician.

MAKING THE RIGHT DECISION ABOUT EMERGENCY CARE

As long as I'm giving advice, I feel compelled to add this section.

If you collapse and are unconscious, or you've been shot, stabbed, run over by a car, or bleeding to death, you don't need my advice. You must get medical care ASAP.

Physicians know the following urgent situations, but too often they go unrecognized by patients, their families, or friends. People, especially the male of the species, will stretch the limits of denial, perhaps until it's too late to avoid death or severe injury.

If you ask, what can be worse than death, talk to survivors of stroke or severe heart disease. Most believed that it "couldn't happen to them."

Heart Attack: If you have crushing chest and left arm pain, break out in a sweat, and you can't breathe, you don't have to be a doctor to know that you'd better head to the ER because it's likely you're having a heart attack. Take note of unusual weakness and sweating even without pain. If you're a woman, you may have instead, "indigestion," jaw or back pain, squeezing discomfort or fullness, or nausea. An early trip to emergency gives physicians the chance to prevent damage from the heart attack or minimize it. Go late, and you may not make it.

Blood Clot to the Lung(s) (Pulmonary Embolism): Sudden shortness of breath, cough, and coughing up blood. Early treatment can save your life.

Stroke: Weakness and/or paralysis are the most obvious symptoms. Sudden, and even transient confusion, dizziness, inability to speak, or sudden blindness should raise the specter of stroke or CVA (cerebrovascular accident). Medical intervention within the first three hours can be life altering to prevent or minimize brain (neurological) damage from a stroke. Sudden extreme headache suggests a subarachnoid bleed. Get to ER immediately.

Asthma: Experts say that nobody should die of asthma, but some do. It's so dramatic that everyone but the most obstinate goes to ER.

Severe Abdominal Pain: On the pain scale 1-10 (the worst), an 8-10 means get to ER ASAP. Such pain strongly suggest one of several abdominal catastrophes.

Incarcerated Hernia: If hernia won't reduce (go back in) with abdominal pain, swelling, nausea and vomiting, it's likely you have a bowel obstruction.

Blood Infection: Fever and shaking chill (teeth chattering, not feeling chilly) suggests sepsis, a medical emergency needing prompt attention.

Spreading Wound Infection: Sores or wounds suddenly becomes painful and spread rapidly.

Irregular or Rapid Heart Beat: Especially associated with weakness, dizziness, or feeling faint may be life-threatening and needs immediate attention.

Some of these trips will prove to be false alarms, but remember the American proverb: Better safe than sorry.

GLOSSARY OF MEDICAL TERMINOLOGY

I did not intend that this glossary will be comprehensive. For that you need to go to *Stedman's Medical Dictionary* or something equally complete. I chose these terms because they appear frequently in the lay literature, even when physicians or other health professionals write them. In my own work, I learned early that it's better to have people understand than to be precise.

abdomen	belly
ablate	to remove or destroy
abrasion	a scrape
aberration	deviation from normal or usual
abscess	a local collection of pus
according to (a person or group)	says (a person or group)
according to (a study)	based on (a study)
accumulation	buildup
acne vulgaris	acne
acquired immune deficiency syndrome	AIDS
acute	sudden or brief
acute abdominal pain	stomachache
acute rhinitis	runny nose; cold (disease)
addictive	habit or dependency forming

adipose	fat
additional	more
administer	give
adolescent	teen
advantage	plus or pro
adverse	harmful or bad
adverse drug reaction	harmful reaction to a drug
affect (noun)	feeling
aggravate	make worse
agitation	restlessness
airway	tubes carrying air to lungs
alcohol dependence	alcoholism
alimentary canal	digestive tract
allergen	allergy-causing substance
allergic rhinitis	hay fever
alleviate	relieve
alopecia	hair loss or baldness
ALS	Lou Gehrig's Disease
alter	change
alteration	change occurred
alternative	choice

amblyopia	loss of sight; no anatomic reason
ambulatory	outpatient or able to walk
ameliorate	improve
amenorrhea	no menstrual periods
analgesic	painkiller
anaphylaxis	severe allergic reaction
anemia	low hemoglobin or red blood cells
aneurysm	dilated or weakened vessel wall
angina	chest pain from heart
angioplasty	balloon repair of narrowed vessel
anomaly	defect
anorexia	loss of appetite
anorexia nervosa	eating disorder with fear of getting fat
anosmia	loss of smell
anoxia	lack of oxygen
anterior	front
anticoagulant	blood thinner
anti-inflammatory	reduces swelling and pain
antipyretic	drug to lower fever
aorta	large artery carrying blood from

	heart
aphthous ulcer	canker sore
apnea	no breathing
appointment	doctor's visit
appropriate	proper
approximately	about
arrhythmia	irregular heartbeat
arterial	artery
arteriogram	x-ray of artery with opaque dye
arteriosclerosis	hardening of the arteries
arthralgia	joint pain
arthritis	joint swelling with pain and tenderness
ascites	fluid in the abdominal cavity
ascorbic acid	vitamin C
aspiration	inhaling a foreign body into lungs
assist	help
association	link
asthma	lung disorder with wheezing
ataxia	walking like a drunk
atherosclerosis	hardening of the arteries

atopic dermatitis	eczema
atrophy	wasting away of body or organ
auditory	hearing or ear
auditory hallucination	hearing things that aren't there
aural	ear
auscultate	listen
autoimmune	immune response to own tissues
autopsy	examination of body after death
axilla	armpit
bacterial	caused by bacteria
beneficial	helpful or good
benign	harmless or not cancerous
benign prostatic hypertrophy(BPH)	non-cancerous prostate enlargement
bereavement	grief
biochemical	chemical
biopsy	tissue sample for diagnosis
bleeding disorder	clotting abnormality
bradycardia	low heart rate
bronchitis	infection bronchial tubes
bruxism	grinding the teeth
bursa	sac around joint for lubrication

caloric expenditure	calories burned
canker	an ulcerous sore
carcinogen	cancer-causing substance
carcinoma	cancer
cardiac	about the heart
carpal tunnel syndrome	nerves in wrist blocked
catheterize	place tube in something, usually the bladder
celiac disease	gluten intolerance
cellulitis	inflammation of tissues
cervical	cervix or neck
characteristic	trait
chemical dependence	addiction
chemotherapy	treating cancer with drugs
cirrhosis	scarred liver from infection or alcohol
clavicle	collarbone
clinician	doctor or therapist
closed comedo	whitehead
cognition	the process of knowing
coitus	sexual intercourse

combination	mix
comedo	acne bump
computed tomography	CT scan or imaging test
conclusion	finding
congenital	inborn or present at birth
congenital anomaly	birth defect
conjunctivitis	pinkeye
consequence	result
contagious	catching
contraception	birth control
contract (a disease)	catch (a disease)
contraindicated	not advised
contrast medium	dye
contusion	bruise
convulsion	seizure or fit
COPD	bronchitis or emphysema
correlation	link
crust	scab
cutaneous	skin
cyanosis	blue color due to insufficient oxygen
debilitating	weakening

defibrillation	shocking the heart to restore heartbeat
deficiency	lack
degeneration	gradual loss or decline
delirium	confusion
delusion	false belief or opinion
dementia	gradual loss of mental abilities
demonstrate	show
depression	Psychiatric despondency
dental caries	tooth decay or cavities
dentition	teeth
dermatitis	rash or skin inflammation
dermatological	about the skin
dermatologist	skin specialist
detect	find
determine	find out
detrimental	harmful or bad
develop (a condition)	get (a condition)
diabetes mellitus	diabetes
diabetic (noun)	person with diabetes
diagnostic procedure	test

dietary	diet
differential diagnosis	list of possible diagnoses
diffuse	widespread
digit	finger or toe
disadvantage	minus or con
dissect	cut apart
disseminated	widespread
disturbance	problem
diverticulitis	inflamed diverticulum in colon
Diverticulum	pouch from wall of the colon
drug dependence	addiction
dysfunction	problem
dysmenorrhea	menstrual cramps
dyspepsia	indigestion
dysphagia	trouble swallowing
dyspnea	trouble breathing
dysuria	painful urination.
echocardiography	heart imaging test
eczema	scaly skin inflammation
edema	swelling
effective	works well

effectiveness	how well (a treatment) works
efficacious	works well
efficacy	how well (a treatment) works
electroconvulsive therapy (ECT)	shock therapy
embolism	material blocking blood vessels
emesis	vomiting
empirical evidence	evidence from experience
endocrinological	gland or hormone
endodontic	root canal
endogenous	inside the person
endometrium	lining of the uterus
enlarge	get bigger
enuresis	lack of bladder control
environment	setting or outside factors
epidermis	outer part of the skin
epidemiologist	expert in disease trends
epidemiology	study of disease trends
epistaxis	bloody nose
epilepsy	having seizures or convulsions
episode	bout or attack
equivalent	equal

erectile dysfunction (ED)	impotence
eruption (skin)	rash or breakout
erythema	redness
establish	set up
etiology	cause
evaluate	assess
exacerbate	make worse
examination	exam or checkup
examine	study or check
excessive	too much
excise	cut out
exhibit	show
exogenous	outside the person
experience (a symptom)	have (a symptom)
experiment	study
experimental	under study
external	outer or outside
extract (a tooth)	pull (a tooth)
exude	ooze
facilitate	make easier
familial	family

fatty acid	fat
febrile	feverish
feces	bowel movement or stool
fibromyalgia	chronic pain around joints
flatulence	gas or fart
flexibility exercise	stretching
Flu	influenza
fracture	break
fructose	fruit sugar
fungal	caused by a fungus
ganglion(cyst)	cystic tumor on tendon sheath
gastric	stomach
gastritis	irritation of stomach lining.
gastroenterologist	digestive disease specialist
gastroesophageal reflux	heartburn
gastrointestinal	stomach and/or intestines
gerontological	age-related
gerontology	science of aging
gestation	pregnancy
glandular	gland
gout	arthritis of small joint, esp. the big

	toe
gynecology	women's health
gynecomastia	enlarged breasts in a man
halitosis	bad breath
hayfever	allergy to plants, grasses etc.
health care facility	hospital or clinic
health maintenance organization	HMO or health plan
hearing impairment	hearing loss or deafness
hearing-impaired	hard of hearing or deaf
heighten	raise
hematological	of the blood
hemorrhage	heavy bleeding
hemorrhoids	enlarge veins around anus
hepatic	liver
heritable	genetic
herpes simplex	cold sore or fever blister
herpes zoster	shingles
heterogeneous	mixed
high-density lipoprotein	HDL or good cholesterol
hirsutism	unwanted hair growth
homogeneous	same or similar

hormonal	hormone
hospitalization	hospital stay
hospice	a place/program for the terminally ill
human immunodeficiency virus	HIV
hypercholesterolemia	high cholesterol
hyperopia	farsightedness
hypersensitivity	allergy
hypertension	high blood pressure
hyperthyroidism	overactive thyroid
hyperventilation	breathing too deeply
hypoglycemia	low blood sugar
hypotension	low blood pressure
hypothyroidism	underactive thyroid
idiopathic	of unknown cause
iatrogenic	caused by the doctor
immunological	immune system
immunotherapy	allergy shots
implement (verb)	carry out
in vitro	in a test tube or lab
incidence	number of new cases
incontinence	lack of bladder or bowel control

indicate	hint or suggest
indicated for	approved or advised for
indication	sign or use
indolent	causing little pain
induration	hardening of body tissue
infantile (condition)	babyhood or childhood (condition)
infectious disease	infection from bacteria, virus etc.
infertility	can't get pregnant
inflammation	redness, swelling, and pain
influence	affect
influenza	flu
ingest	eat or drink
ingestion	intake
inhibit	limit or block
initiate	start
injection	shot
inpatient facility	hospital
insomnia	trouble sleeping
insulin	hormone controlling blood sugar
intermittent	on-again, off-again
internal	inner or inside

intervention	treatment
intramuscular	in a muscle
intravenous	IV or in a vein
investigate	study
investigational	under study
in situ	in the body
in vitro	in the lab
ischemia	insufficient oxygen supply to an organ
jaundice	yellow-looking skin
juvenile (condition)	childhood (condition)
kidney stones	stones in urinary system
kyphosis	humpback
laboratory	lab
laceration	cut
lactation	breast-feeding
lactose	milk sugar
larynx	voice box
lesion	sore or wound
lethargic	sluggish, tired
leukemia	blood cancer producing white cells

limb	arm or leg
lingual	tongue
lipid	fat or fat-like substance
localized	around the (body part)
location	site
lordosis	inward curvature of spine
low-density lipoprotein	LDL or bad cholesterol
lupus	antibodies against own tissues
macule	discolored skin spot
magnetic resonance imaging	MRI or imaging test
major depressive disorder	depression
malaise	feeling ill
malignant	cancerous
malignant melanoma	cancer of a mole
malingering	faking illness
malocclusion	overbite or underbite
mammary	breast
management (of a disease)	control (of a disease)
mandible	lower jaw
manifestation	sign or symptom
maximal	maximum

mean (statistical)	average (statistical)
medication	drug
medicolegal	medical and legal
meningitis	infected membranes around brain
menses	menstrual period
menopause	periods end. Estrogen deficiency.
metastasize	spread
migraine	severe recurring headache, one-sided
miliaria	prickly heat
mitral valve prolapsed	floppy mitral valve
mobility	ability to get around
moderate (verb)	limit
modify	change
monitor	track
morbidity	disease rate
mortality	death rate
motility	movement
multipara	two or more children
multiple	many
muscular	muscle
musculoskeletal	muscles and bones

mutation	genetic defect
mycotic	caused by a fungus
myocardial infarction	heart attack
myopia	nearsightedness
nasal	nose
nausea	upset stomach
neonate	newborn
neoplasm	tumor or growth
neuralgia	nerve pain
neurological	brain and/or nervous system
neuron	nerve cell
nevus	mole or birthmark
nocturnal enuresis	bed-wetting
nodule	lump
obese	overweight
obstruct	block or close
occlude	block or close
occlusion	blockage
occupational	job-related
ocular	eye
olfactory	smell

oncological	cancer
oncologist	cancer specialist
onset	start
open comedo	blackhead
ophthalmological	eye
ophthalmologist	eye specialist
optimal	best
orally	by mouth
organization	group
orthodontia	braces
osteoporosis	thinning of the bone
otalgia	earache
otitis externa	outer ear infection
otitis media	middle ear infection
otorhinolaryngologist	ear-nose-throat specialist
outpatient facility	clinic
ovum	egg
palliate	to relieve without curing
palliative	giving relief but not curing
pallor	paleness
palpate	feel by hand

palpitation	feeling rapid or irregular heartbeat
pancreatitis	inflammation of pancreas
panic attack	nervous disorder: rapid breathing
papule	bump (skin)
Parkinson's disease	neurologic tremor and rigidity
participate	take part
parturition	labor and delivery
patella	kneecap
pathogenesis	how a disease develops
pathognomonic	characteristic of a disease
patient	person
pediatric	childhood or children's
pediculosis	lice, crabs
penile	penis
peptic ulcer	ulcer
perforate	make a hole in
perform	do
periodontist	gum disease specialist
periodontitis	gum disease
perioral	around the mouth
peritoneal cavity	abdominal cavity

persist	last
persistent	long-lasting
perspire	sweat
pertussis	whooping cough
pervasive	wide-ranging
pharmaceutical	drug
pharyngeal	about the throat
pharyngitis	sore throat
pharynx	throat
phototherapy	light therapy
physician	doctor
physiological	bodily
pigmentation	color
placebo	sugar pill
plaque (artery)	fatty deposit
plasma	blood
plasma glucose	blood sugar
podiatric	foot
pneumonia	infection in the lung.
podiatrist	foot doctor
positron emission tomography	PET scan or imaging test

posterior	back
postoperative	after surgery
postprandial	after a meal
practitioner	doctor or therapist
preadolescent	preteen
preclinical	not yet causing symptoms
predisposed (to)	prone (to)
predisposition	tendency
preferred provider organization	PPO or health plan
premalignant	abnormal, but not yet cancerous
preoperative	before surgery
present with	have
prevalence	total number of cases
prevalent	common
preventative	preventive
primary	main
principal	main
principal investigator	head researcher
probability	odds
prognosis	outlook
progressive	gets worse with time

prone(position)	lying on your stomach
prophylaxis	preventive or protective treatment
pruritus	itching
psoriasis	skin disease with scaling
psychological	mental
psychomotor	mental and physical
psychoneuroimmunology	mind-body link
psychopathology	mental illness
psychopharmacologist	psychiatrist prescribing medication
psychosis	loss of contact with reality
psychosocial	mental and social
psychotherapy	therapy
psychotropic	mind-altering
ptosis	drooping, esp. of eyelid
pulmonary	lung
purpura	bruising
purulence	pus
purulent	filled with pus
pustule	pimple
radiation	x-rays
recommendation	tip or advice

recur	return
recurrence	return
recurrent	repeated
reduction	loss or decline
reduction(fracture)	put back in place
refractory	hard-to-treat
referral	sending you to another doctor
relapse	slip or backslide
renal	kidney
renal failure	kidneys not working to eliminate waste
resistance training	strength training or lifting weights
respiration	breathing
respondent (in a survey)	person (in a survey)
retardation	slowing down
retinol	vitamin A
rubella	German measles
rubeola	measles
rupture	burst
scale (skin)	flake
scapula	shoulder blade

scoliosis	lateral curvature of spine
seborrheic dermatitis	dandruff or cradle cap
secondary to	due to
sedentary	inactive
seizures	convulsions, fits
self-management	self-care
senile (condition)	age-related (condition)
senile dementia	Alzheimer's/other related dementias
senile lentigo	liver spot
sinusitis	infected sinuses
skeletal	bone
skin tag	extra skin flesh, benign
sleep apnea	stopping breathing during sleep
smoking cessation	quitting smoking
sodium chloride	salt
somnambulism	sleepwalking
specimen	sample
spontaneous abortion	miscarriage
stabilized	holding steady
staphylococcal	staph
STD	sexually transmitted disease

stenosis	narrowing
stent	frame to keep vessel open
sternum	breastbone
strabismus	cross-eye
streptococcal	strep
stridor	noise breathing from blocked airway
stroke	paralysis from blocked vessel or bleed
subcutaneous	just under the skin
subject (in research)	person or volunteer (in research)
sucrose	table sugar
sufferer from (a disease)	person with (a disease)
suggestion	tip or advice
supervision	guidance
supine	lying on your back
susceptible (to)	prone (to)
suture	sew up or close
symptomatology	symptoms
syncope	fainting
synthetic	man-made
systemic	whole-body

systemic lupus erythematosus	lupus
tactile	touch
tachycardia	rapid heart beat
tarsal	ankle
tendonitis	inflammation of a tendon
terminal	is going to die
testicular	testicles
testis	testicle
therapeutic modality	therapy or treatment
thoracic	chest
thrombolytic therapy	clot-dissolving drug
tibia	shinbone
tinea corporis	ringworm
tinea cruris	jock itch
tinea pedis	athlete's foot
tinnitus	ringing in the ears
TMJ	temporomandibular joint
tonsillitis	infection of tonsils
topical application	applied to the skin
toxic	poisonous
toxin	poison

trachea	windpipe
transient ischemic attack (TIA)	ministroke
transmission	spread
transmit (a disease)	spread (a disease)
transplantation	transplant
trauma	injury
tremor	shaking
ulcer	sore
ultrasonography	ultrasound or imaging test
URI	upper respiratory infection
UTI	urinary tract infection
urticaria	hives
uterus	womb
vaccine	to prevent infectious disease
variable	factor
varicella	chickenpox
varicose veins	enlarge veins in lower extremity
vascular	blood vessel
vasculitis	inflammation of blood vessel
venous	vein
venous thrombosis	clot in vein

ventricular fibrillation	chaotic heart beat
verruca	wart
vertigo	dizziness
vesicle	blister
victim of (a disease)	person with (a disease)
viral	caused by a virus
viscera	internal organs
visual hallucination	seeing things that aren't there
visual impairment	vision loss or blindness
void	urinate
vulnerable (to)	prone (to)
zoonosis	disease spread from animals to people

MEDICAL SPECIALISTS

Allergist or Immunologist: diagnosis and treatment of allergic conditions.

Anesthesiologist: administers anesthesia and monitors the patient during surgery. Pain control.

Cardiologist: diagnose and treat heart disease

Cardiovascular surgeon: operates on heart and great blood vessels.

Colorectal Surgeon: operates on colon, anus, and rectum.

Clinical Geneticist: diagnose and treat genetic disorders.

Critical Care Specialist: cares for patients in intensive care units.

Dermatologist: treats skin diseases and skin cancers

Endocrinologist: disease of endocrine glands, esp. diabetes.

Forensic Pathologist: coroners and medical examiners.

Gastroenterologist: treats stomach and intestinal disorders

Geriatrician: treats disease of age.

Gynecologist: treats female reproductive system and genital tract.

Hematologist: treats diseases of the blood and blood-forming tissues

Hepatologist: diagnose and treat diseases of the liver.

Hospitalist: treats patients in the hospital in place of primary care physicians.

Infectious Disease Specialist: Diagnoses and treats infectious diseases.

Internal Medicine Physician: prevention, diagnosis, and treatment of adult diseases.

Nephrologist: treats kidney diseases.

Neurologist: diagnoses and treats diseases and disorders of the nervous system.

Neurosurgeon: operates on the nervous system.

Nuclear Medicine Specialist: uses imaging techniques to diagnose diseases.

Nurse-Midwifery: woman's health care during pregnancy, delivery, and the postpartum period.

Obstetrician: treats women during pregnancy and childbirth

Occupational Medicine Physician: diagnoses and treats work-related disease or injury.

Oncologist: diagnoses and treats cancer.

Ophthalmologist: treats eye defects, injuries, and diseases.

Oral and Maxillofacial Surgeon: surgically treats diseases, injuries, and defects of the hard and soft tissues of the face, mouth, and jaws.

Orthopedic Surgeon: surgical treatment of joints, fractures.

Otolaryngologist: treats diseases of the ear, nose, and throat, and head and neck.

Pathologist: examines body tissues for diagnosis.

Pediatrician: treats infants, toddlers, children and teenagers.

Physiatrist: Physical medicine and rehabilitation.

Plastic Surgeon: restores, reconstructs, corrects or improves the appearance of body structures.

Podiatrist: provides medical and surgical treatment of the foot.

Psychiatrist: treats patients with mental/emotional disorders.

Pulmonary Medicine Physician: diagnoses and treats lung disorders.

Radiation Oncologist: diagnoses and treats cancer and other disorders with radiation.

Diagnostic Radiologist: diagnoses and medically treats diseases with imaging techniques.

Rheumatologist: treats arthritis and autoimmune diseases.

Urologist: diagnoses and treats urinary tract and the male reproductive system.

www.ingramcontent.com/pod-product-compliance
Lightning Source LLC
Chambersburg PA
CBHW081356280526
45788CB00009B/2898
9781523837250